DEBORAH SHANNON

Strength Training For Seniors

Easy to Follow Strength, Flexibility, and Balance Exercises

This book was professionally typeset on Reedsy.
Find out more at reedsy.com

Contents

1

Introduction

Welcome to Strength Training for Seniors! I am Deborah Shannon, and I have taught circuit fitness classes for seniors at our gym since 2019. This short book introduces a few workout routines I teach to help seniors and younger people build strength, balance, flexibility, and endurance. These workouts are designed to keep you motivated and engaged while working on different body parts each time.

Resistance training is an effective way to build stronger muscles and denser bones. It can be done using dumbbells or simply by using your body weight. It is essential to pace yourself during the workout and prioritize safety and comfort. If any exercise causes pain or discomfort, please stop immediately and consult with your healthcare professional.

Each person has their own fitness goals and limitations. Therefore, modifying these workout routines to make them less or more intense, depending on your fitness level, is essential. I encourage people to listen to their bodies and do what feels right.

This book will work on strength, balance, flexibility, endurance, proper breathing, and hydration. We will have two routines, and the third will be putting those two routines together, which takes about 45 minutes. You can try doing these routines two or three days a week, resting a day in between workouts. If using weights, they should challenge you while keeping good form.

What to Expect

The workout begins with a warm-up that can be done either sitting on a sturdy chair or standing next to or behind it. The warm-up includes marching, shoulder rolls, waist rotations, calf raises, and leg raises.

After the warm-up, we move on to the lower body workout, which includes marching, alternate knee raises, chair squats, and leg raises. The workout also has modifications for each exercise, so you can choose the one that suits you the best.

The workout ends with a balance exercise of standing on one leg without holding onto the chair.

Remember to take water breaks whenever needed and breathe appropriately during each exercise. You can also listen to your favorite music while working out to make it more enjoyable. Let's get exercising and have fun! I like to change the workouts so no one gets bored and work on different body parts at other times. However, I will only include a few workout routines for this book. I aim to get you up and moving and have fun doing it!

I also suggest that you pace yourselves so you can finish your workout. Always prioritize safety and comfort. If any exercise causes pain or discomfort, please stop.

Feel free to do two or three sets of each routine. Why not try doing these two or three days a week, resting a day in between workouts? Also, if using weights, they should challenge you while keeping good form.

Before Starting Your Workout

- Have two dumbbells of either two, three, or five lbs. or two water bottles to use as weights.
- Wear comfortable clothing and shoes
- Have drinking water available
- Have enough space to move around comfortably.

Are you Ready? Let's Get Exercising!
Why not play some music? I love the 60's oldies!
HAVE FUN!

2

Warm Up

You can be seated in your sturdy chair or stand next to/or behind it

Let's inhale through your nose and exhale through your mouth. Try not to hold your breath while exercising, and take a water break whenever needed.

March:

- Stand with your feet hip-width apart.
- March in place while pumping your arms, maintaining good posture.
- March for about 30-60 seconds

Don't forget to breathe!

Shoulder Rolls:

- Sit or stand with your arms hanging loosely at your sides.
- Roll your shoulders circularly, moving them forward for a few rotations.
- Reverse the direction and roll them backward.
- Perform 8-10 rotations in each direction.

Waist Rotations:

- Space your feet hip distance apart
- Stretch your arms out to the side, hold your core tight, and rotate at the waist to the right and then to the left.
- Repeat eight times

Calf raises:

- Stand behind your chair or sit
- Lift heels up and down
- Perform ten times

Leg Raises:

- Stand next to your chair or sit
- Lift one leg straight before you, keeping it straight but not locked.
- Lower the leg and repeat with the other leg.
- Perform 8-10 leg raises on each leg.

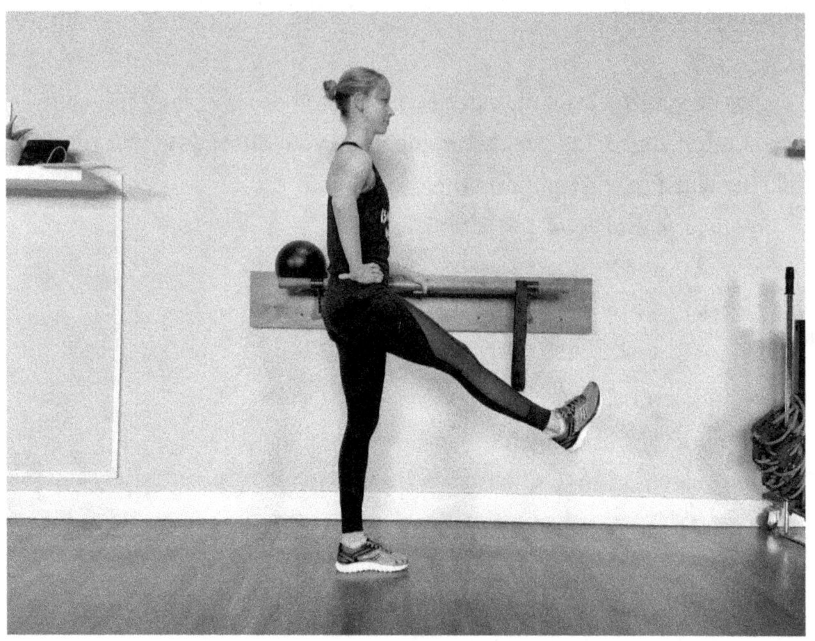

Deep breathe in and exhale.
  Water break

3

Lower Body Workout

March and pump arms for 30 -60 seconds

Alternate knee raises:

- Sit or Stand with feet shoulder-width apart
- Alternate raising knees
- Repeat ten times.

Modification:

- Sit and slightly raise your knees, alternating legs
- Stand and raise your knees higher than a 45-degree angle for a *greater challenge*

Water if needed

Chair squats:

- Begin by sitting on the forward part of your chair; feet should be directly below your knees, hip distance apart, and good posture should be maintained while sitting.
- Push down on your heels, put hands on your thighs, or extend them out front for balance, engage your core, and stand.
- Repeat ten times.

Modification:

- Push down on your heels, put your hands on your thighs or the side of the chair, and start to stand by lifting off the chair a *few inches.*
- Or, push down on your heels and tighten your quad and glute muscles.
- Hold a weight under your chin to add *more challenge.*

Water if needed

Leg Raises:

- Sit in your chair with good posture. Lift one leg straight before you, keeping it straight but not locked.
- Lower and raise the leg ten times
- Repeat with the other leg.

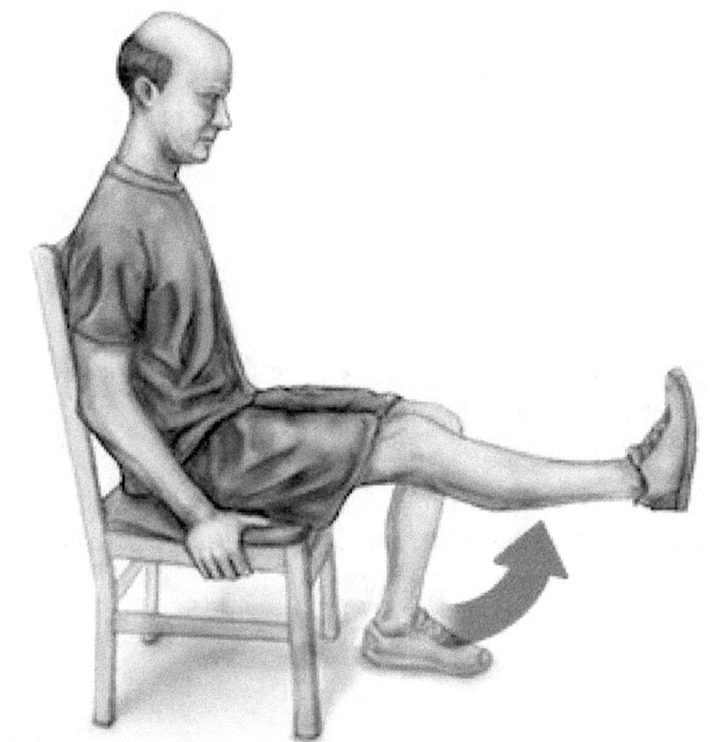

Sitting Leg Raise

Modification:

- Lower the leg slightly so it is below the waist height, and do smaller movements and fewer reps.
- Hold one weight on the thigh near your knee to *add resistance* and perform the exercise.

Water break
  Deep breathe in and exhale

Knee raises:

- Stand or sit with good posture
- Raise one knee (waist high or higher) and lower 12 times
- Repeat with the other leg.

Modification:

- Sit and minimize movement
- Hold one weight on the thigh near the knee to add resistance and perform knee raises.

Water break

REPEAT THIS UPPER BODY ROUTINE ONE OR TWO MORE TIMES WHEN YOU ARE READY FOR MORE!

4

Balance

- Stand tall next to or behind your chair, shoulders up, back, and down.
- Hold the back of the chair while shifting all of your weight onto one leg.
- Slowly bend the other knee slightly so your foot is hovering over the floor.

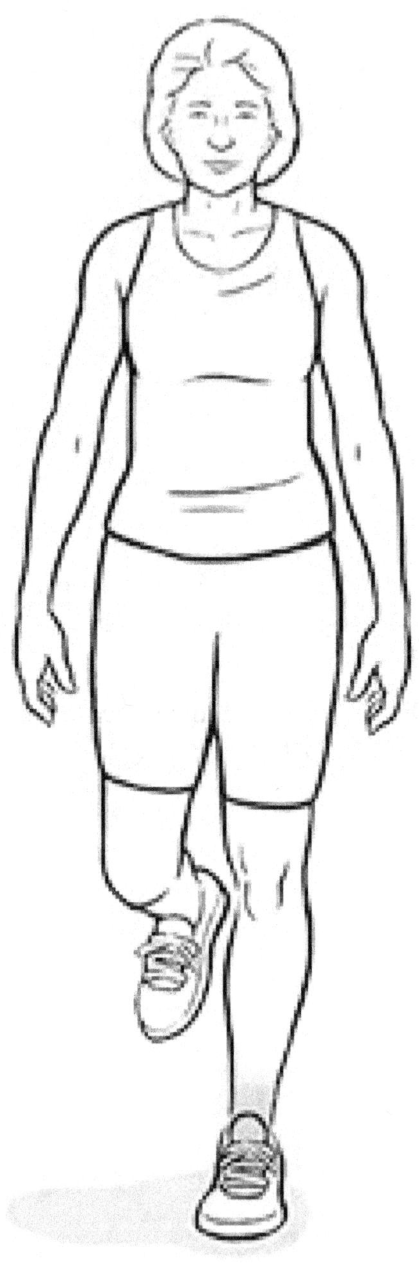

- Fun balance challenge: Slowly release your hand from the chair or most fingers. Feel all of those stabilizer muscles working. Feel your big toe and little toe working.
- Can you hold this for 30 seconds or longer?

- It helps to focus your eyes on one thing and not look around.
- Rest and repeat with the other leg.

Balance exercises are something to work on every day. Think about balancing while you're waiting for your tea or coffee. The counter is right there if you need to hold on.

5

Cool Down

- Sit in your chair. Take a deep breath in and exhale slowly. Repeat one more time.
- Extend one leg out front, heel on the floor, and toe up toward the ceiling.
- Inhale and exhale while hinging forward at the waist to feel that nice stretch in the hamstring muscle. Inhale and exhale again. Hold for 30 seconds.
- Repeat with the other leg.
- Sit up. Rotate your shoulders frontwards eight times and backward eight times.
- Shrug 4 times
- Deep breath in and exhale slowly.
- Inhale and exhale while turning your head left and hold for a few seconds. Return front, inhale, exhale while turning your head to the right, and hold for a few seconds—return facing front.
- Take a deep breath while raising your arms, and exhale while

lowering your arms.
- Clap your hands and applaud yourself for completing the lower body routine!!

CONGRATULATIONS! YOU DID IT! I AM SO PROUD OF YOU!

Continue to the Upper Body Workout or rest a day

Upper Body Workout

Go straight to the workout if you are continuing from the lower body workout.

Please refer to the warm-up section before continuing the upper body workout if you rested for a day.

Take a few deep breaths and remember to drink water whenever needed. Also, If you need to stop during an exercise, please do it and then get back into it. **You can do this!**

Bicep Curls:

- Sit or Stand with feet shoulder-width apart
- Hold dumbbells or a water bottle in each hand

- Put your arms down at your sides, elbows tucked near your waist, palms facing up.
- Inhale
- Engage your core, exhale, bend your elbows while keeping them at your side, and raise the weights to the chest.
- Inhale and lower the weights back to the starting position
- Repeat 10–12 times

Modification

- Perform these exercises without weights
- Increase the weight of your dumbbells for a *more challenging* workout

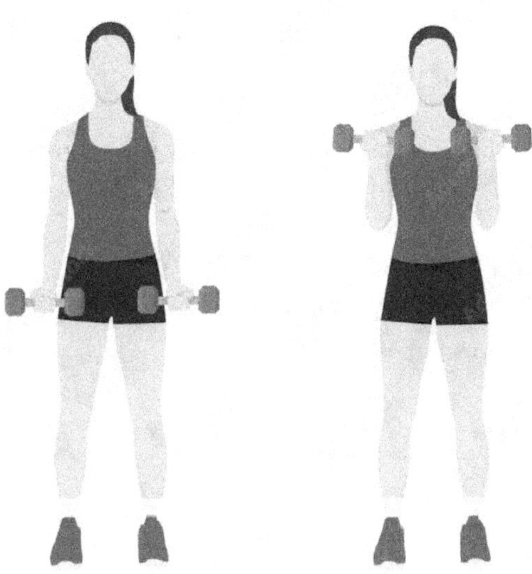

Water Break

Tricep Extensions

- Sit or stand with feet shoulder-width apart
- Hold one weight in each hand
- Slightly bend your knees (if standing) and hinge forward at the hips while keeping your back straight.
- Arms should hang down with palms facing each other.

- Engage your core, inhale, and bend your elbows to a 45-degree angle
- Exhale and straighten your elbows, and extend the weights behind you
- Hold for a moment
- Bend the elbows and return to the starting position.
- Repeat 10-12 times

Modification

- Perform these exercises without weights
- Increase the weight of your dumbbells or increase the reps for a *more challenging* workout

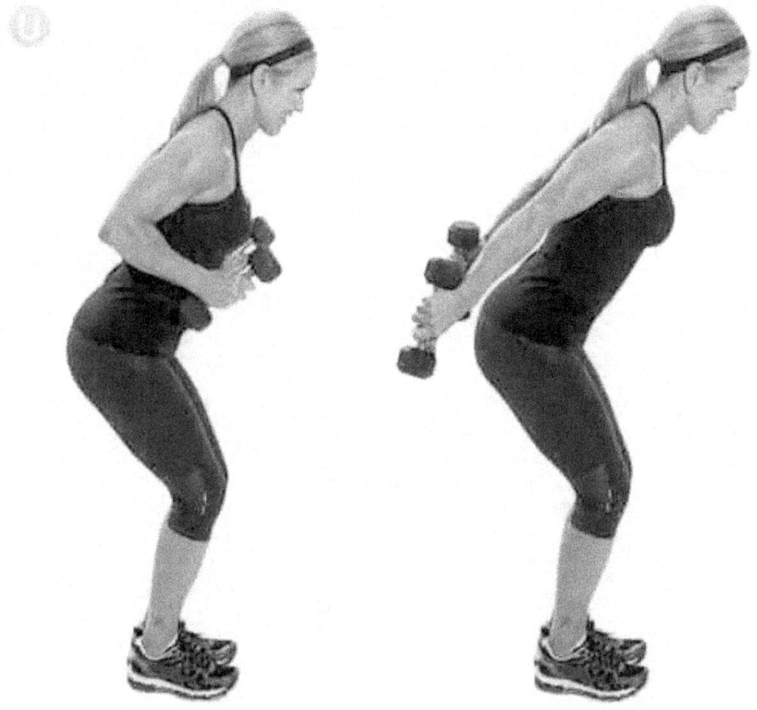

Water Break

Overhead Press

- Stand or sit with good posture
- Hold a dumbbell or water bottle in each hand, arms at your side, palms facing each other.
- Inhale and bend your elbows
- Exhale and raise your weights overhead (try to straighten your elbows)
- Inhale and lower the weights while bending your elbows
- Return to starting position
- Repeat 8-12 times

Modification

- Perform these exercises without weights
- Increase the weight of your dumbbells or increase the reps for *more challenge*

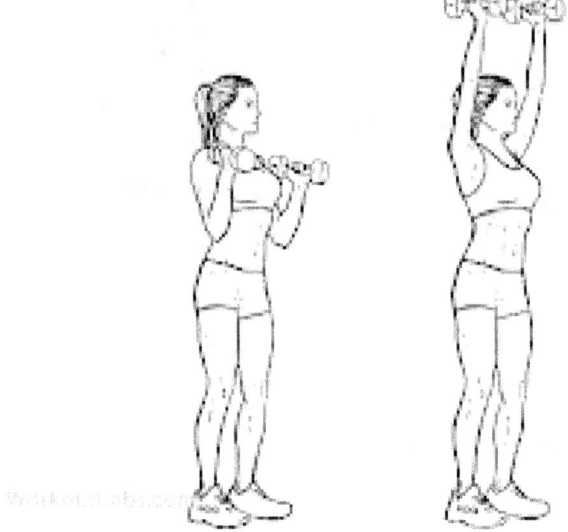

Water break

Work your way up to doing 2 to 3 sets of these upper body routines.
Balance

- Perform the balance routine again

Refer back to the cool-down section of this book
I am so proud of you! You did a fantastic job!

6

Full Body Workout

- Start from the warm-up and perform the lower body workout, the upper body workout, and the balance routine.
- Repeat 2-3 sets

Continue onto the cool down.

Drink plenty of water

Congratulations again! You are amazing!

Conclusion

Thank you, all, for exercising with me. My goal is to be as strong, fit, and independent as possible. I hope this will become your goal as well.

Please remember that consistency matters. Keep moving. Yesterday is gone. Today is what matters! God bless you all!

Deborah